You Are Not Your Trauma Healing Journal:
40 Days to Reclaiming Self & Writing New Chapters

HARRIET M. HARRIS, MBA

Copyright © 2024 Harriet M. Harris, MBA

All rights reserved.

www.harrietmharris.com

No part of this book may be reproduced or transmitted in any form or by any means, electronic or mechanical, including photocopying, recording, or by any information storage and retrieval system, without permission in writing from the copyright owner.

Disclaimer: Disclaimer: This book is not a substitute for therapy. The information within is not intended to guarantee healing in any way. Its purpose is to provide tools to understand, identify and work through traumatic experiences to begin to see your life in a renewed way. If you need additional support and guidance, please seek the assistance of a professional coach or therapist.

Printed in the United States of America
ISBN: 979-8-9873578-1-1

DEDICATION

"And we know that in all things God works for the good of those who love him, who have been called according to his purpose." - Romans 8:28

Most of my life, I felt overshadowed by trauma, uncertain and hurt, almost believing I was too broken for God to use. Yet, through His grace, that very journey of struggle transformed me into a woman chosen to guide others through their valleys. I am deeply grateful to those who stood by me during my darkest moments, often unaware of my silent battles.

To my incredible parents and brother, your support in the depths of my struggle, even when it was hard to understand, was my anchor. Your unwavering love and strength in my weakest moments are a testament to God's unconditional love. To my children, you are my 'why' — the very essence of the future I desire to brighten. Your existence propelled me to heal and lead by example, to show you that even in our darkest moments, God's love and purpose shine through.

To my husband, thank you for your patience and love, even when my fears and pain cast a shadow over us. For all the love you've given, even when I was lost in my fears, thank you. Your support has been a crucial part in my healing journey.

Each of you have journeyed with me from the shadows into the light, witnessing my growth from suffering in my pain to finding my purpose. I couldn't have embarked on this path without your love and support. Thank you for being part of my story, a story that tells a powerful truth: our past does not define us, it's how we rise from it that truly shapes our narrative. I thank God for placing you in my life. I dedicate this book to you:

Keidrick Harris, Sr.
Keidrick Harris, Jr.
Camden Harris
Kayleigh Harris
Harry McInnis
Pamela McInnis
Jarvis McInnis

CONTENTS

PREFACE 7
ACKNOWLEDGMENTS 11
INTRODUCTION 13
UNDERSTANDING TRAUMA 15
UNDERSTANDING WHAT TRAUMA ISN'T? 23
PART 1: AWAKENING 45
PART 2: EXPLORATION 67
PART 3: TRANSFORMATION 89
PART 4: BLOSSOMING 111
AFTER THE 40 DAYS 132
CHARTING YOUR PATH FORWARD 137
ABOUT THE AUTHOR 171

PREFACE

In the heart of every shadow lies the potential for an immense light – the foundational belief that inspired the creation of this book. My journey, which may be similar to yours, has included periods of darkness, moments where trauma seemed to define every part of my existence. I have wrestled with my fair share of shadows, navigating the intricate dance of darkness, pain, healing, and understanding. While shadow work is undeniably crucial, a question lingered: What comes next?

This book was written based on the realization that while facing our shadows is crucial, there's more to the journey than just looking back. The real challenge lies in finding the courage to look forward again—or maybe or the first time. You may be asking yourself, "How do I envision a brighter future when my past experiences have clouded my vision and dimmed my spirits?" The key is to start by acknowledging the impact of those experiences, while recognizing that they do not define your entire journey. For too long, many of us have felt trapped in our past, unable to see a way out, let alone a path forward. But by embracing healing and growth, you can begin to see beyond the pain and towards a future filled with hope and new possibilities.

You Are Not Your Trauma isn't just a title, it's a movement- a truth I learned to embrace and want to share with you. This book isn't just about understanding your past – it's also about taking back control of your story and writing a new chapter, one where trauma informs but does not control your destiny.

Over the next 40 days, through guided journaling, introspective prompts, and reflective exercises, this journal invites you to begin a journey of transformation. Each page is an opportunity to explore what has been and what can be. It's a journey from acknowledging the pain to embracing the growth beyond it.

The purpose of this book is to guide you in rewriting your future story — a story liberated from the chains of past trauma. It's about discovering a life where your experiences are your strengths, where each day is a step towards a new, empowering narrative.

So, I invite you to take this journey and step into the light that awaits you beyond the shadows.

MESSAGE FROM THE AUTHOR

Greetings fellow survivor,

I want to say how incredibly proud I am of you for taking this step. Starting a healing journey isn't easy, but you're here, and that's huge. I'm cheering you on every step of the way.

Healing from trauma can be tricky—I've been there myself. When I started my journey, it felt like I was meeting a whole new me for the first time.

That journey of self-discovery and raw vulnerability sparked something in me. I felt this urgent need to share my story, to let others know that healing is possible, and you don't have to stay stuck in the pain. I wanted to be living proof that there's still light, even in our darkest moments. That inspired me to start You Are Not Your Trauma™ podcast.

But talking wasn't enough. I wanted to create something tangible that could walk alongside you on your healing journey. And that's where this journal comes in. It's my way of reaching out and helping you reclaim your joy and authentic self.

Over the next 40 days, this journal will guide you on your own journey of self-discovery. Don't think of it as just another book—but like a friend there to hold your hand through it all. This book is your sacred, safe space where you can meet yourself with kindness and understanding and rewrite your story with courage and grace, one day at a time.

So, as you fill these pages with your heart and your dreams, remember there are no rules here. You can scream, dream, cry, and rediscover your resilient spirit.

I'm here with you, cheering you on as you create the chapters of your life waiting to be written with hope, resilience, and self-love.

Be brave, be kind to yourself, and remember that every day is a chance to embrace who you are a little more.

With warmth and solidarity,

Harriet M. Harris, MBA

ACKNOWLEDGMENTS

First and foremost, I thank God for guiding me on this journey and helping me find purpose in one of the most difficult experiences of my life.

A heartfelt thank you to my family and friends for your unwavering support as I journeyed through my healing process. Your love, encouragement, and belief in me have been my anchor, giving me the strength to move forward and embrace a brighter future.

To my mentors, thank you for your wisdom and encouragement. Your guidance has profoundly shaped my approach to healing.

A special thanks to the designer of my cover for bringing beauty and warmth to these pages, making this journal not just a tool for reflection but a comforting companion.

And to you, the reader and writer of your own story, thank you for trusting this journal as a space to explore, heal, and grow. Your journey is a testament to the strength and resilience of the human spirit. May the pages you fill serve as a reminder of your progress and inspire your continued journey.

Thank you from the bottom of my heart for being an essential part of this journey. Here's to the chapters yet unwritten and the stories you'll continue to tell.

With deepest gratitude,

Harriet M. Harris, MBA

Introduction

Welcome to the start of your journey toward reshaping your story and discovering what's possible beyond the trauma. This book will guide you through reflection, healing, and growth with a mix of thoughtful reading and guided journaling—helping you move forward with clarity and strength, one step at a time.

In many spiritual traditions, including biblical context, the period of 40 days is considered a sacred and transformative time — a period of renewal, rediscovery, and growth. It symbolizes times of change, preparation, and transition. From the 40 days and nights Moses spent on Mount Sinai to Jesus' 40 days in the wilderness and the 40 days of Lent, this timeframe encourages reflection, transformation, and renewal.

You are about to begin a powerful 40-day journey, where you'll start reshaping your story with resilience, renewal, and growth. This is your time to reconnect with your true self, move beyond the pain of past experiences, and rediscover the vibrant person within you—full of dreams, strength, and endless possibilities.

You hold the pen in this significant chapter of your life, where you begin to reshape the stories shaped by trauma. As the author of your own journey, the canvas is yours to fill with the vibrant colors of growth, change, and new dreams.

In this journal, you will take a 40-day journey guided by specifically crafted prompts, each offering a stepping-stone to writing your new chapters. They will gently reconnect you with your true self, offering spaces to dream, hope, and envision a future crafted meticulously with words of strength, resilience, and joy.

Through each day's reflection and writing, see yourself as a gardener nurturing a plot of land, investing love, time, and energy, watching new buds grow, and witnessing the transformation daily until a beautiful garden of vibrant experiences, dreams, and narratives unfold before you.

Let these 40 days be a sacred space where you redefine your story, claim your right to dream and hope, and build a future aligned with the person you aspire to be. Step by step, day by day, you will uncover new parts of yourself and begin creating a life full of fresh experiences and perspectives —no longer defined by the trauma that once held such a significant place in your story.

Here's to you, the courageous soul embarking on this 40-day journey to reclaim yourself and take control of your story, shaping it with hope, dreams, and new possibilities.

Welcome to your new beginning, a space where every word you write becomes a testament to your resilience and a step towards a future crafted by you for you.

Understanding Trauma

Navigating the twisted paths of healing personally, I've come to realize that understanding trauma is essential on the journey to rediscover oneself. Trauma has a cunning way of embedding itself in the nooks and crannies of our soul, operating in silence, subtly influencing our thoughts and actions from the shadows. The critical task at hand is not to let trauma become the puppet master of our existence. If we don't confront our trauma, it begins to dictate our narrative, steering us from a place of pain and vulnerability rather than one of strength and growth.

Trauma is indeed a complex and multifaceted beast, often residing in the depths of our psyche, subtly affecting our lives in myriad ways. Many of us encounter trauma, yet fully understanding its depths, its intricate nuances, and its pervasive impacts remains a challenge. To truly grasp what trauma entails, embark on a journey of deep discovery and self-awareness. It requires us to untangle the web of our experiences, to recognize and differentiate the various forms it takes, and to understand how it shapes our perceptions, relationships, and choices.

This journey of understanding begins with acknowledging that trauma is often more than the immediate reactions to a distressing event. It can manifest in lingering feelings of anxiety, in unexpected moments of panic, in the sudden onset of fear, and even in places where we once felt safe. The effects of trauma might surface in our relationships, where we find ourselves reacting intensely to seemingly minor issues or struggling to form deep, meaningful connections. It might show up in our body, where unprocessed trauma can manifest as physical pain, fatigue, or other somatic symptoms.

Understanding trauma also means recognizing its role in shaping our belief systems and self-identity. It can lead us to view the world through fear and distrust, question our self-worth, or feel powerless to change our circumstances. Uncovering these layers of trauma involves - peeling back the narratives we've told ourselves, examining the beliefs we've held onto, and challenging the limits we've placed on ourselves.

Beyond these personal impacts, trauma can have broader societal implications. It can be generational, passed down through family dynamics, cultural narratives, or societal structures. Recognizing this helps us see our trauma not just as a personal struggle but as a part of a larger tapestry of human experience, one that connects us with others in our vulnerabilities and strengths.

The ultimate goal in understanding trauma is not to erase its existence but to diminish its control over our lives and learn to navigate its presence with awareness, compassion, and resilience. This process involves developing strategies to cope with the immediate effects of trauma, such as mindfulness, grounding techniques, and therapeutic interventions. It also means building a support system that includes professional help and nurturing relationships that offer understanding, acceptance, and encouragement.

As we begin to understand and heal from trauma, we begin to reclaim our narrative. We move from a place of being reactive to our experiences to one where we are actively reshaping our story. We learn to recognize our triggers, to soothe our pain, to celebrate our growth, and to find joy in our journey. In doing so, we transform our relationship with our past and, in turn, open up new possibilities for our future.

What is Trauma?

Think of trauma as the emotional earthquake that shakes up your world when something too big, too scary, or just too much for your mind to handle happens. It's like a deep cut in your psychological makeup, messing with your head and heart in ways that go beyond just feeling scared or upset. Trauma sticks around, becoming this unwanted guest in your thoughts, changing how you see and interact with the world.

Unfortunately, it doesn't just fade away—instead, it hangs around, making you feel like you've lost a part of yourself. You might end up feeling all adrift, caught in a whirlpool of emotions that don't make sense, feeling vulnerable in ways that stop you from connecting with people or enjoying the simple things in life.

Trauma is sneaky too. It's not just about those big, dramatic moments. Sometimes, it's the smaller things that chip away at you over time. It can come from anywhere – a crash, being sick for a long time, harsh words that stick, trusting someone who lets you down, saying goodbye to someone you love, being abused, sexually assaulted, or even realizing a truth that turns your world upside down. These experiences dig in deep because of what they mean to you.

The aftermath? It's like dropping a stone in water – the ripples keep spreading. Trauma can make you jumpy, always on edge, like you're waiting for the next bad thing to happen. It can mess with your sleep, make you snappy, scatter your focus, and even show up as aches and pains. Your body and brain are always on high alert, making everything else much harder.

And let's talk memory – trauma can have you re-living the worst moments over and over, so vivid it's like you're right back there. Or it might make you want to avoid anything that reminds you of those times, making holes in your memory to keep the pain at bay.

Understanding trauma helps you see how it turns your world upside down and accept that healing isn't a straightforward path. Healing is a journey of facing those harsh memories, questioning old ways of thinking, and, piece by piece, finding your way back to feeling safe and whole.

Trauma is Personal

Coming to terms with just how personal trauma is can be a game-changer for those who have experienced trauma as well as those who have not. Trauma wears many faces and hits everyone differently – it's as unique to each person as their fingerprint, molded by their life's story, beliefs, and lived experiences. What shakes one person might roll right off another. Embracing this uniqueness is critical to honoring your healing journey and removing the idea that there's only one way to heal.

For some, a job loss might shake their world to its core, while for others, it's a tough bump in the road they feel equipped to handle. Neither reaction is less valid than the other; they just show how varied our experiences of trauma can be.

And here's the thing—trauma isn't about how big the outside world perceives an event to be—it's more about how big the impact feels to you. Whether it's one monumental event or a string of stressors, if it rocks your well-being, it counts.

How you react to a traumatic experience is totally valid, no matter what it looks like. From numbness and denial to anger or intense sadness, all the ways our minds and bodies try to cope with trauma's heaviness make sense. Some of us pull back, and some of us are on high alert all the time – it's all part of the complex dance of getting through.

Healing from trauma? That's a personal journey, too. There's no one-size-fits-all remedy. Whether it's talk therapy, somatic therapy, diving into creative outlets, finding solace in community, or seeking peace through spirituality, the "best" way to heal is the way that feels right to you.

By really understanding how personal trauma is, we open up a world where healing is about empathy, patience, and walking your own path. You will want to surround yourself with people who are willing to lend an ear without judgment, offer a shoulder without assumptions, and, above all, respect the individual journey you will navigate.

Everyone who experiences trauma will have their own unique experience, and it will be up to them how they choose to face it.

The Many Faces of Trauma

Let's talk about how trauma isn't a one-size-fits-all kind of deal. It's more like a spectrum, with a range of experiences affecting people in wildly different ways. Understanding this can change the game in how you tackle healing.

On one end, you've got the big, life-upending stuff—things like surviving a natural disaster, being sexually assaulted, experiencing violence, or losing someone you love suddenly. These events can knock the wind out of you, leaving scars that might lead to something like PTSD. They're the kind of experiences that can turn your world upside down, affecting everything from how you feel inside to how you connect with others.

Then, there's the stuff that might not make the evening news but can shake you up just as much. I'm talking about the experiences that stick with you—being bullied, going through a tough breakup, or facing rejection. These moments might seem "smaller" on the surface, but they pack a punch emotionally and psychologically, shaping how you see the world and yourself.

The reality is trauma doesn't care about how big or small an experience looks from the outside. It's more about what it feels like on the inside. Something that seems manageable to one person can be earth-shattering to another. It's super personal, influenced by your past, how you cope, and who's in your corner.

Recognizing trauma's versatility helps us see the complete picture. People can face different kinds of trauma, sometimes all at once or one after another, each layer adding to the weight of the other. It's a complex mix that affects everyone uniquely, needing a healing touch that's just as personalized.

This way of seeing trauma opens our hearts wider. It teaches us to meet each other's stories without judgment, understanding that there's no single story of what trauma looks like. It reminds us that healing isn't a straight path but a journey that looks different for everyone, demanding patience, kindness, and a tailor-made approach.

So, as we navigate our paths or stand beside others on theirs, let's remember the many faces of trauma. Let's offer our hands, ears, and hearts, ready to support each other in finding the way through in all the ways that matter.

Stepping Into Healing: Your Journey of Transformation

Kicking off your healing journey is HUGE! Seriously, applaud yourself for even considering this leap. The journey you are about to begin will be about peeling back the layers of your trauma, truly seeing yourself—bruises and all—and saying, "Yeah, I'm still standing." The road won't be smooth, it will be scattered with hurdles and heartaches, but believe me, it will also include moments of sheer brilliance, growth, and deep, deep self-revelation.

Healing isn't about pretending specific chapters of your life didn't happen. Nope, it's more about taking the knowledge from those chapters to decide how to write the future chapters, changing the tone from pain to power, from victim to survivor. It's about highlighting your resilience, self-love, and ability to find strength even in difficult circumstances.

Facing trauma is tough. There's no doubt about that. It forces you to sit in the storm, feel every drop of pain, hurt, anger, and disappointment, and then gradually find a way to move forward. It's a process of slowly releasing trauma's grip on your life, ensuring that you are the one in control, steering towards your aspirations rather than being driven by fear.

As you stand at the brink of your journey, ready to dive in, remember the fire inside you. You've got this incredible resilience, a warrior spirit ready to wrestle with the shadows and come out into the light as you begin to understand yourself in ways you never realized you needed to.

And hey, walking this path doesn't mean you're walking it alone. There are people out there, guides and fellow survivors, ready to walk with you. Support is a big piece of this puzzle, whether it's a therapist who gets it, support groups that feel like home or just friends and family who offer their hearts and ears.

Every little step you take is a declaration that you're more than your past, that your story is still being written and has chapters filled with light, love, and laughter ahead. So, take a deep breath, my friend, and step into this journey, ready to write the next chapter of your story with every word and every moment of courage. You are not your trauma— you're a whole universe waiting to unfold, and it's time to start turning the pages and creating new possibilities.

Understanding What Trauma Isn't

As you navigate through understanding trauma, it's just as essential to get clarity on what trauma isn't. It's not a badge of dishonor or a shadow that chains down your entire being. And it's not a label you're stuck with or a dark cloud that permanently hangs over you.

Let's bust some myths and clear the air around trauma:

It's Not Your Fault: Let this sink in deep. Trauma leaves many feeling guilty as if they somehow invited it. But hear this loud and clear: you are not to blame for the storms that came your way. The circumstances leading to trauma were out of your control, and you carry no fault for the hurt you've endured.

It Doesn't Mean You're Weak: There's this wrong idea floating around that if you're traumatized, you're somehow less tough. That's a myth that needs to be kicked to the curb. Making it through trauma, day by day, shows a kind of strength that's monumental. True strength isn't about never feeling down. It's about keeping on despite the heavy hits.

It Doesn't Define You: Sure, trauma is a big deal, and it shapes parts of your life, but it's not all you are. You're this amazing, complex person with your own mix of stories, thoughts, feelings, and dreams. Your past troubles are just one part of who you are.

It's Not an Overreaction: Whatever you're feeling after trauma—those emotions are valid. It's okay to feel hurt and express what's inside without holding back. These feelings are natural responses to something that was too much to bear.

It Shouldn't be Ignored: Trying to ignore trauma or pretend it's not a big deal is like pressing down on a spring- it's going to bounce back harder. Facing your trauma head-on is the way through it. Keeping silent only makes the healing road longer and bumpier. One thing for certain, if you don't deal with your trauma, it will deal with you. And it won't be nice about it or gentle with you. But by confronting it, you're taking back your power and choosing to heal and deal on your terms.

It Doesn't Seal Your Fate: While trauma might influence some chapters of your life, it doesn't get to write the whole book. You've got the power to shape your story as you move forward. The future is a canvas still in your hands, ready for the new dreams you want to paint on it.

Understanding what trauma isn't paves the way for healing while removing the stigma attached to trauma. With that clarity, you can see trauma for what it really is, just a chapter in the story of your life. You have the strength, the courage, and the heart to move beyond trauma and take control of the narrative moving forward.

Why You Are Not Your Trauma

Trauma will convince you that it's the main character in the story of your life. It can make you feel as if it's the lens through which everything else is viewed, overshadowing all the other parts that make you who you are. It's like walking through life with a shadow that follows you everywhere, casting darkness over your identity and making it difficult to see the light of your own essence. In the thick of it, it's all too easy to forget that you are so much more than the chapters of hardship.

Your journey through trauma, as significant as it is, is just a part of a much larger, richer narrative that is your life. It doesn't capture all of you. Think of yourself as a garden, flourishing with various flowers—laughter, successes, dreams, relationships, struggles, and losses. Each piece adds to the beauty of your garden, with trauma being just one not-so-beautiful flower among many. It's shaped you, sure, but it's not the only thing that has.

You've got a name, a heart full of dreams, things that make you light up, and love that runs deep. And guess what? These parts of you didn't disappear when trauma showed up. You wear many hats—friend, maybe lover, sibling, or parent. You've felt joy, those moments that make your heart do a happy dance, like when laughter bubbles up uncontrollably or when everything just clicks into place. Those bursts of joy are like splashes of color on the canvas of your life, adding depth and vibrancy to your story.

The emotions trauma brings up—fear, anger, deep sadness—they're not signs of weakness. They're signs of being human, of having a heart that feels deeply, even when things get tough. Your ability to feel those emotions and keep pushing forward? That's strength and resilience right there.

Even when it doesn't feel like it, remember this: you're capable of growth and transformation beyond your trauma. Humans are amazing at healing, learning, and finding strength, even in the messiest situations. You have the power to write new chapters in your life, ones filled with recovery, personal growth, and fresh starts.

Every step you take is a step towards reclaiming your identity, stepping out from the shadows of trauma into the brilliance of your true self. It's a journey of recognition and celebration—of seeing yourself, possibly for the first time in a long while, and embracing the full spectrum of who you are, including the resilience and hope that's always been part of your story.

You are Not Defined by Your Bad Experiences

It's easy to think of trauma as being the headline track of your life's playlist, playing on repeat and overshadowing every other song that makes up your soundtrack. It's easy to feel like those intense, painful moments are the only tunes defining you, like they're the only tracks that matter. But here's the real deal: your life's playlist is richer and more varied than just a single song of trauma.

Focusing only on the trauma tunes can drown out the rest of your music. For every song of sorrow, there's a whole album of tracks filled with strength, joy, and perseverance. Think about the times you've bounced back stronger, the unexpected happy moments that have lifted you, the resilience you've shown, and the positive vibes you've spread. These are your anthems, just as defining of who you are.

It's possible to remix how you see your life, not as a single on repeat but as an ever-growing album. This new view allows you to see trauma as just one song among many in your collection. You're the DJ here, with the power to decide which tracks get airtime and how you want to blend them into your life's soundtrack.

Embracing your life's playlist is empowering. It increases the volume of the possibilities for your future, where your past tracks don't have to define your next releases. Each day is an opportunity to add new songs to your playlist, expanding the soundtrack of your life. Your past may have set your playlist's foundation, but the next tracks are yours to choose and play.

You Have Unseen Strength

Battling through trauma might make you feel like you're constantly fighting a losing battle. But here's a truth bomb for you: in the midst of all that chaos, you've tapped into a well of strength you probably didn't even know existed. We're talking about a deep, powerful kind of grit that doesn't always make a grand entrance with fanfare. Instead, the quiet resolve that whispers in your ear, "Keep pushing forward," even when forward seems like a foreign concept.

Imagine being in the middle of an emotional hurricane, where every wave of memory and every gust of pain seems determined to knock you down. And yet, here you are, still standing, still fighting. It's not just luck or fate. It's a testament to your unseen strength. The kind of inner strength that doesn't always shout from the rooftops but is there, steady and unwavering, guiding you through the storm.

This strength I'm talking about? It's the backbone of your spirit, the part of you that refuses to be crushed under the weight of your experiences. It enables you to face the darkest nights and still hold onto the sliver of hope that daylight is coming. It's in how you adapt, pick up pieces, figure out new ways to cope, and reach out when isolation feels like the easier choice. This determination has been your silent partner, carrying you through when you feel alone.

Redefining strength is also important. Real strength isn't about never feeling down or scared, but about feeling all those things and deciding to keep going anyway. There is bravery in your vulnerability, courage in asking for help, and boldness in taking even the smallest steps toward healing.

Being able to recognize your unseen strength is powerful. It reframes your story from a narrative of victimhood to one of victory and courage. It's a reminder that, within you lies an extraordinary ability to heal, grow, and start fresh. This strength is your ally, quietly asserting, "You are more than your trauma. You are a survivor, a warrior, and your journey is far from over."

Your unseen strength is waiting to be acknowledged, nurtured, and celebrated. It's time for you to see just how powerful you really are.

You are Who God Says You Are

Navigating through the aftermath of trauma can feel like losing a piece of yourself, leaving you adrift in a sea of confusion and pain. But here's a truth to anchor you: your true identity isn't tethered to these storms. As a child of God, you're rooted in something far more profound and enduring than life's tumultuous moments. You're defined by God's unwavering and affirming words, not by the shifting sands of circumstance.

Think of it this way—you're part of a chosen lineage, as 1 Peter 2:9 highlights. You're not just a face in the crowd, YOU are royalty, handpicked and cherished in God's eyes. I'm not talking about wearing a physical crown kind of loyalty, but about embracing the dignity, value, and purpose that result from being God's child. You carry a light within you that no darkness can dim.

Jeremiah 31:3 talks about everlasting love—an unconditional, unending kind of love that surpasses our understanding. It gives us a glimpse of our true worth through God's eyes. Even when we feel lost or unworthy, this promise of eternal love is a lifeline that you can hold on to during life gets hard, it should remind you that you are deeply cherished.

The image of being held in God's hand speaks volumes about protection and care. It symbolizes a safety and security that the world can't provide, an assurance that, despite the chaos, you are protected by the Almighty. This assurance isn't just for calm moments but shines brightest in the midst of adversity, offering peace and hope.

Embracing your identity as God's child, will transform how you perceive yourself and your journey. It's a shift from seeing yourself as a casualty of life's battles to recognizing yourself as a conqueror in Christ. It's understanding that your worth and direction aren't dictated by past hurts but by God's loving declarations.

You Can Rediscover Your True Self

Setting out to rediscover yourself takes guts and faith because it's not easy. You will have to peel back all the layers of pain and fear left by trauma to uncover the real you – the person God intended you to be, with unique gifts, potential, and purpose. Your journey won't be just about healing, it'll also be about transforming yourself, getting back in touch with your true self, and aligning with God's plan and purpose for your life.

Realizing that your trauma doesn't define your identity is the crucial first step. It opens up a whole new world where you can explore, grow, and redefine yourself beyond past hurts. This process involves digging deep into your soul, questioning the beliefs and stories you've told yourself, and letting go of the ones that have kept you stuck. Allowing you to shed the false identities trauma may have imposed on you and embracing the truth of who you truly are.

The next step is living out that truth in your daily life by actively choosing to honor your worth, and staying true to your authentic self, even when it's tough. It means making decisions that align with your newfound understanding of yourself and not letting past pain dictate your present and future.

As you walk this path, you'll face challenges and triumphs. There will be moments of doubt, fear, insight, and joy. Every step forward, no matter how small, will bring you closer to understanding yourself better, reconnecting with your inner strength, and reigniting the dreams that may have faded.

This journey is also about recognizing and embracing the unique purpose God has for you and realizing that your experiences, even the painful ones, have shaped you into someone with empathy, resilience, and wisdom. Your journey can inspire others and show them that healing and growth are possible.

You're not alone on this journey. God is by your side, offering love, guidance, and strength every step of the way. And you'll find others walking a similar path, ready to support and encourage you too.

The journey of rediscovering yourself is one of the most important you'll ever take. It leads to healing, growth, and a more profound sense of purpose. So, get ready to write new chapters in your life story filled with hope, resilience, and the rediscovery of the incredible person God created you to be.

You Have the Power to Shape Your Future

In the story of your life, you're not just a character – you're the primary author. This empowering truth is what must propel you forward on your journey. Despite the challenges and setbacks that trauma may have thrown your way, you still hold the pen. You have the remarkable power to decide your future and create a story that reflects your dreams, values, and the wisdom you've gained along the way.

Embracing this power means also embracing that your past doesn't dictate your future. Yes, the chapters marked by trauma are significant, but they don't have the final say. You get to write new chapters filled with hope, joy, and purpose. Nothing can erase the past, nor should the impact of your experiences be downplayed, instead, integrate those experiences into your story in a way that allows you to move forward.

As the author of your story, you're free to dream and pursue a future that excites you. It may involve setting fresh goals, reigniting dormant passions, or nurturing relationships that lift you up. It could mean shedding old habits and beliefs that no longer serve you and replacing them with ones that empower you to flourish.

In shaping your future, lean on the divine wisdom and love surrounding you. Whether through prayer, meditation, or seeking counsel from trusted mentors and friends, tap into the guidance and support available to you as you chart your course ahead.

Now, be prepared because shaping your future isn't a one-time deal, it's an ongoing journey of growth and adaptation. You will have to make choices every day that align with the person you aspire to be and the life you desire to live. While you can't control everything that happens, you always have the power to choose how you respond and what steps you take next.

You have the power to mold your future, turning your experiences – even the painful ones – into stepping stones for growth and transformation. You're actively writing your story with each decision, action, and thought—a story that's uniquely yours, full of resilience, hope, and the promise of brighter days ahead.

You Are Not Broken—Embrace You

Moving forward in your journey of healing and self-discovery is not about denying or erasing the traumatic events that have shaped you but about embracing your whole self—the pain and the strength, the hurt and the healing. It's crucial to acknowledge that while your traumatic experiences are a part of you, they do not encompass all that you are or all that you can be. Embracing your whole self means accepting your past and understanding its impact but also recognizing the vast potential for growth, wisdom, and resilience within you.

Trauma, undoubtedly, can leave deep scars, but it also has the potential to cultivate an incredible depth of wisdom and empathy. The experiences you've been through can give you unique insights into the complexities of life and the human spirit. They can heighten your ability to connect with others who are suffering, offering comfort and understanding rooted in genuine experience. Wisdom that can only come from walking through the fire and emerging, not unscathed, but stronger and more compassionate.

Resilience is another gift that often emerges from healing from trauma. The quiet strength that enables you to face each day, even when you carry the weight of your past with you. Having resilience doesn't mean you will never frustrated or overwhelmed, it means that you have the ability to dig deep and find the courage to keep going when you have to —to take one more step, even when the path is uncertain. It's a testament to your ability to endure and to find ways to thrive under challenging circumstances.

Grace is the another key component in embracing your entire self. It involves extending kindness and understanding to yourself, forgiving yourself for not having all the answers, and accepting that it's okay to not always feel strong. While we often show kindness to others, we may neglect to do the same for ourselves. Therefore, treating ourselves with the same compassion and gentleness that we would offer to a friend in pain is critical as we navigate our own journey's.

Pre-Journal Activity: Honoring Your Story

Before you dive into this journey of healing and rediscovery, take some time to honor and acknowledge the path you've walked so far. This pre-journal activity is a sacred space for you to gently and safely confront the traumas that have shaped your life. It's a moment to pause and recognize the challenges you've faced, setting the stage for your journey of healing.

Remember, this is **YOUR** personal space, and there is no obligation to share it with anyone.

Instructions:

1. **Find a Quiet Space**: Ensure you are in a comfortable, quiet space where you won't be disturbed. Take a few deep breaths, grounding yourself in the present moment.

2. **Prayer or Meditation**: If it aligns with your beliefs, begin with a prayer or a moment of meditation. Seek strength and guidance for the journey you are about to undertake. Ask for courage, wisdom and compassion as you remember your past experiences.

3. **List Your Traumas**: Turn to the next few pages and start listing the traumas or traumatic experiences that have impacted your life. You might write these as words, phrases, or even brief descriptions. Name each trauma in a way that feels authentic to you. Approach this task with kindness towards yourself, recognizing that you don't need to capture every detail if it feels overwhelming.

4. **Emotions and Sensations**: Beside each listed trauma or traumatic experience, write down the emotions and physical sensations that accompany it. This could range from feelings of anxiety, sadness, or anger, to physical responses such as tension, fatigue, or discomfort. Acknowledging these feelings and sensations is a way of validating your experience.

5. **Your Safe Symbols**: At the end of your list, choose a symbol, word, or phrase that embodies safety and healing for you. It might be a verse

from scripture, a personal mantra, or a visual symbol like a calm ocean or a sturdy oak tree. Draw or write this symbol as a personal emblem of your commitment to healing.

6. **Closing Ritual**: Conclude this activity with a self-care ritual. This could be something simple yet comforting, such as wrapping yourself in a cozy blanket, enjoying a warm cup of tea, or reading an inspiring passage. This ritual is a way of nurturing yourself and setting a protective, compassionate tone for your journey.

Note:

- **This is Your Journey**: Remember that this is your journey, and you determine the pace. It is perfectly okay to take breaks or to do this activity over several days.

- **Seek Support When Needed**: If at any point this activity becomes overwhelming or triggers deep pain, don't hesitate to reach out to a supportive friend, family member, or a trauma informed professional.

****

The 40-Day Journey Ahead

After documenting your traumas or traumatic experiences, you're set to begin the 40-day journey toward healing, growth, and rediscovery. Each day will bring guided prompts, reflective exercises, and affirmations to help you reconnect with the joyful, resilient, and beautiful individual you are – the person God created you to be. Through this process, you'll work to reclaim yourself and your narrative, creating new chapters filled with hope, strength, and self-compassion.

As you proceed, remember this is a journey toward healing, a path where traumas do not define you but rather serve as stepping stones towards recovery, growth, and the full realization of God's grace in your life. Each step you take is a move towards embracing your whole self, shedding the weight of the past, and stepping into a future filled with promise and light.

How to Use the Journal

This journaling journey is a powerful step towards discovering or rediscovering the beauty and potential that life still holds. This journal is your guide to recognizing and embracing the richness of your life, beyond your experiences of trauma.

1. **Recognize Your Starting Point**: Begin by acknowledging your current state. It's completely normal if trauma overshadows other aspects of your life at this stage. Embrace your feelings as valid and understand that acknowledging where you are now is a brave first step on your path forward.
2. **Focus on Growth and Possibility**: Each prompt in this journal is designed to help you shift your focus from past to present and future. As you respond, concentrate on the strengths you've developed, the lessons you've learned, and the dreams you still cherish.
3. **Daily Affirmations**: At the end of each journaling session, you'll find an affirmation. These are potent words that affirm your potential and the unchanging positive aspects of life, no matter what your past entails. Repeat these affirmations, believe in their truth, and let them be your guide.
4. **Visualize a Bright Future**: With each entry, allow yourself to visualize a life beyond trauma. Picture the endless possibilities that await – the places you'll explore, the joy you'll find, and the growth you'll experience.
5. **Prioritize Healing Over Re-living**: While processing trauma is important, the aim of this journal is to focus on healing. Use your writing to guide your thoughts towards recovery, resilience, and growth, rather than dwelling on past events.
6. **Shift the Lens**: If your focus drifts back to traumatic experiences, gently guide your thoughts back to growth and forward movement. Ask yourself, "How does this reflection contribute to my journey ahead? What can I learn from it to propel me towards a brighter future?"
7. **Celebrate Life Daily**: Commit to recognizing and celebrating life's joyful moments, however small. Cherish a moment of laughter, a personal achievement, or a connection with someone or something that brings you happiness.
8. **Seek Support When Needed**: If the journey of looking

forward feels daunting, don't hesitate to seek support from trusted individuals, support groups, or professionals equipped to assist you in navigating these emotions.
9. **Reflect and Act**: Use your reflections as a foundation for action. Set small, achievable goals that align with your vision for the future, and take steps towards realizing them.
10. **Document Your Journey**: Keep a record of your thoughts, feelings, and changes in perspective. This log will be a testament to your evolution, showcasing how you've shifted your focus from past to future.

Remember, this journey is about shedding light on your path forward, recognizing the fullness of your life and its potential. As you work your way through the pages, it will be a reminder that while trauma is part of your story, it isn't the whole story. Let this journal be your compass in navigating the rich landscape of your life.

In You Are Not Your Trauma Healing Journal, the goal extends beyond just surviving to thriving. I want you to be able to envision a life beyond trauma and tap into your inner strength to make that vision a reality. Trust in this process, believe in your immense potential, and remember: each new page is your opportunity to write a chapter filled with hope, resilience, and growth.

Welcome to your transformative journey!

Navigating Emotions: Daily Mood Tracking

As you navigate through your journal each day, you'll be using a special tool at the end of your entries: the Daily Mood Tracker, paired with the Feel Wheel. Now, you might ask, "Why a wheel?" Here's the thing – sometimes we feel off or just not quite right, and we can't put our finger on why. That's where the Feel Wheel spins into action.

It's easy to get stuck on the surface of our emotions, like saying we're just "fine" or "stressed." But if we dig a little deeper, we often find there's more to our mood. The Feel Wheel helps us do just that. It breaks down those broad, sometimes vague feelings into more specific emotions. Maybe what we thought was just stress is actually a mix of frustration, disappointment, or even anticipation.

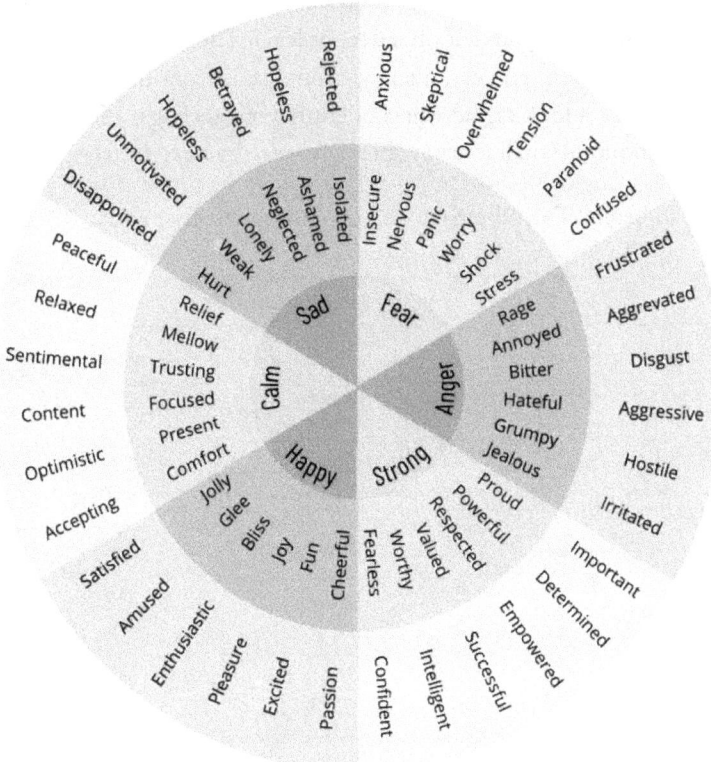

Using the Feel Wheel, you can pinpoint the exact emotion you're feeling. Consider it as a map for you to use when you're not sure where you are – it gives you a starting point to understand your emotional state better. Each day, after you jot down your thoughts and reflections, look at the Feel Wheel. See where your mood lands and track it. Over time, you'll start to see patterns and get to know your emotional landscape a lot better.

I don't want you to think of this of just tracking your mood, instead see it as a way to get to know yourself on a deeper level. The better you understand your emotions, the more you can manage them, learn from them, and ultimately grow. So, take a look at the wheel, identify your feelings, and map out the feelings and emotions you will journey through during the next 40 days.

Ready to start? Turn the page, and dive into your first entry.

I don't want you to think of this as just tracking your mood; instead, see it as a way to get to know yourself on a deeper level. The better you understand your emotions, the more you can manage them, learn from them, and ultimately grow. So, take a look at the wheel, identify your feelings, and start mapping out the emotions you'll journey through over the next 40 days.

Ready to begin? Turn the page and dive into your first entry.

Part 1: Awakening

(Days 1-10)

Awakening to Your Inner Strengths

As you start this journey, the first step is about waking up to the amazing strengths you already have inside you. Think of this as laying the groundwork for the big changes that are coming your way. With each day's prompts, try to gently tune into what's already inside you. It's like turning on a light to see all the great qualities and abilities you've got, which will guide you on this path of discovering more about yourself and starting anew.

1. Picture the first day of your new chapter. What does it look like? Feel like?

Example: On the first day of my new chapter, I wake up feeling rested. I have a healthy breakfast and spend some time in the garden, enjoying the quiet.

_____
_____
_____
_____
_____
_____
_____
_____
_____
_____
_____
_____
_____
_____
_____
_____
_____
_____
_____
_____
_____
_____
_____
_____
_____
_____
_____
_____

YOU ARE NOT YOUR TRAUMA HEALING JOURNAL

Confident	Excited	Calm	Appreciated	Afraid	Hurt	Angry
Determined	Happy	Content	Loved	Alarmed	Lonely	Annoyed
Encouraged	Hopeful	Focused	Supported	Anxious	Sad	Frustrated
Proud	Optimistic	Mindful	Valued	Fearful	Upset	Irritated
Supported	Overjoyed	Peaceful		Nervous		Mad
	Positive	Relaxed		Worried		

Notes_____

I am open to new beginnings.

2. Think about the times in your life that really stand out, the ones that you want to shape your story, apart from any traumatic experiences.

Example: The day I graduated, the first time I successfully led a team project, and the day I decided to start therapy.

_____
_____
_____
_____
_____
_____
_____
_____
_____
_____
_____
_____
_____
_____
_____
_____
_____
_____
_____
_____
_____
_____
_____
_____
_____
_____
_____
_____
_____
_____
_____
_____

YOU ARE NOT YOUR TRAUMA HEALING JOURNAL

Confident	Excited	Calm	Appreciated	Afraid	Hurt	Angry
Determined	Happy	Content	Loved	Alarmed	Lonely	Annoyed
Encouraged	Hopeful	Focused	Supported	Anxious	Sad	Frustrated
Proud	Optimistic	Mindful	Valued	Fearful	Upset	Irritated
Supported	Overjoyed	Peaceful		Nervous		Mad
	Positive	Relaxed		Worried		

Notes _____

I choose the moments that define me.

3. Think of your life as a big library, what would you name the next three books (or chapters) in your story?

Example: Book One: 'Recovery Road,' Book Two: 'Strength Unleashed,' Book Three: 'Adventures in Serenity.'

YOU ARE NOT YOUR TRAUMA HEALING JOURNAL

Confident	Excited	Calm	Appreciated	Afraid	Hurt	Angry
Determined	Happy	Content	Loved	Alarmed	Lonely	Annoyed
Encouraged	Hopeful	Focused	Supported	Anxious	Sad	Frustrated
Proud	Optimistic	Mindful	Valued	Fearful	Upset	Irritated
Supported	Overjoyed	Peaceful		Nervous		Mad
	Positive	Relaxed		Worried		

Notes_____

I am the author of my future chapters.

4. As you consider to your new chapters, think about the strengths you hold within. Which of these strengths are going to take center stage in your life's new story? And how do you envision using them to shape your journey or healing and growth?

Example: One of my key strengths is resilience. I plan to let this resilience lead the way in my new story, using it to stay strong and hopeful, even when things get tough.

YOU ARE NOT YOUR TRAUMA HEALING JOURNAL

Confident	Excited	Calm	Appreciated	Afraid	Hurt	Angry
Determined	Happy	Content	Loved	Alarmed	Lonely	Annoyed
Encouraged	Hopeful	Focused	Supported	Anxious	Sad	Frustrated
Proud	Optimistic	Mindful	Valued	Fearful	Upset	Irritated
Supported	Overjoyed	Peaceful		Nervous		Mad
	Positive	Relaxed		Worried		

Notes_____

My strengths are the heroes of my story.

5. Think about a recent experience you've had. How could you look at in a way that displays any personal growth or resilience, even if it's just a little bit?

Example: Last week I was criticized at work, but instead of getting defensive, I used it as an opportunity to improve.

Confident	Excited	Calm	Appreciated	Afraid	Hurt	Angry
Determined	Happy	Content	Loved	Alarmed	Lonely	Annoyed
Encouraged	Hopeful	Focused	Supported	Anxious	Sad	Frustrated
Proud	Optimistic	Mindful	Valued	Fearful	Upset	Irritated
Supported	Overjoyed	Peaceful		Nervous		Mad
	Positive	Relaxed		Worried		
☐	☐	☐	☐	☐	☐	☐

Notes _____

I am viewing my experiences through a lens of growth and resilience.

6. Imagine you've already gotten past this tough chapter of trauma. What would that stronger, healed version of yourself say to you at this moment?

Example: You've already come so far, and you're just getting stronger. Keep going!

YOU ARE NOT YOUR TRAUMA HEALING JOURNAL

Confident	Excited	Calm	Appreciated	Afraid	Hurt	Angry
Determined	Happy	Content	Loved	Alarmed	Lonely	Annoyed
Encouraged	Hopeful	Focused	Supported	Anxious	Sad	Frustrated
Proud	Optimistic	Mindful	Valued	Fearful	Upset	Irritated
Supported	Overjoyed	Peaceful		Nervous		Mad
	Positive	Relaxed		Worried		

Notes_____

I listen to and honor the wisdom of my inner champion.

7. Think back to a time recently when you felt really happy out of the blue. How can you create more happy moments in the new chapters of your life?

Example: Hearing an old favorite song on the radio unexpectedly made me smile and dance in the kitchen. To enjoy more moments like this, I plan to make a playlist of feel-good songs to brighten my daily routine.

YOU ARE NOT YOUR TRAUMA HEALING JOURNAL

Confident	Excited	Calm	Appreciated	Afraid	Hurt	Angry
Determined	Happy	Content	Loved	Alarmed	Lonely	Annoyed
Encouraged	Hopeful	Focused	Supported	Anxious	Sad	Frustrated
Proud	Optimistic	Mindful	Valued	Fearful	Upset	Irritated
Supported	Overjoyed	Peaceful		Nervous		Mad
	Positive	Relaxed		Worried		

Notes_____

I embrace and celebrate spontaneous joy in my life.

8. What are some ways you can bring little moments of peace and happiness into your everyday life on purpose?

Example: Starting my day with a ten-minute meditation seems to set a positive tone for me.

Confident	Excited	Calm	Appreciated	Afraid	Hurt	Angry
Determined	Happy	Content	Loved	Alarmed	Lonely	Annoyed
Encouraged	Hopeful	Focused	Supported	Anxious	Sad	Frustrated
Proud	Optimistic	Mindful	Valued	Fearful	Upset	Irritated
Supported	Overjoyed	Peaceful		Nervous		Mad
	Positive	Relaxed		Worried		

Notes _____

I have the power to cultivate peace and happiness in my life.

9. When you were a kid, what were some of the dreams or things you really wanted to do when you grew up?

YOU ARE NOT YOUR TRAUMA HEALING JOURNAL

Confident	Excited	Calm	Appreciated	Afraid	Hurt	Angry
Determined	Happy	Content	Loved	Alarmed	Lonely	Annoyed
Encouraged	Hopeful	Focused	Supported	Anxious	Sad	Frustrated
Proud	Optimistic	Mindful	Valued	Fearful	Upset	Irritated
Supported	Overjoyed	Peaceful		Nervous		Mad
	Positive	Relaxed		Worried		

Notes

I honor the dreams and aspirations of my youthful self.

10. Write a letter to your future self, the one you'll be a year from now. In this letter, pour out all your hopes, dreams, and plans for where you want your life's story to be. What do you want to tell your future self about the journey you're hoping to embark on?

_____
_____
_____
_____
_____
_____
_____
_____
_____
_____
_____
_____
_____
_____
_____
_____
_____
_____
_____
_____
_____
_____
_____
_____
_____
_____
_____
_____
_____
_____
_____

Confident	Excited	Calm	Appreciated	Afraid	Hurt	Angry
Determined	Happy	Content	Loved	Alarmed	Lonely	Annoyed
Encouraged	Hopeful	Focused	Supported	Anxious	Sad	Frustrated
Proud	Optimistic	Mindful	Valued	Fearful	Upset	Irritated
Supported	Overjoyed	Peaceful		Nervous		Mad
	Positive	Relaxed		Worried		
☐	☐	☐	☐	☐	☐	☐

Notes _____

I trust in the journey and the path I am crafting for myself.

Part 2: Exploration

(Days 11-20)

Diving Deeper into Your Inner Self

Now's the time to really dive deep and explore the hidden corners of your inner world. Approach this next phase with curiosity and an open heart. This is your chance to get up close and personal with what you truly want, what scares you, and what you dream about. Use this time to weave a story for yourself that's filled with self-compassion and an appreciation of your own complexities.

11. As you continue exploring the depths of who you are in this phase, think about any songs, poems, or quotes that really speak to the story you're trying to create for yourself. Why do these particular words or melodies strike a chord with you?

YOU ARE NOT YOUR TRAUMA HEALING JOURNAL

Confident	Excited	Calm	Appreciated	Afraid	Hurt	Angry
Determined	Happy	Content	Loved	Alarmed	Lonely	Annoyed
Encouraged	Hopeful	Focused	Supported	Anxious	Sad	Frustrated
Proud	Optimistic	Mindful	Valued	Fearful	Upset	Irritated
Supported	Overjoyed	Peaceful		Nervous		Mad
	Positive	Relaxed		Worried		
☐	☐	☐	☐	☐	☐	☐

Notes_____

I am inspired and guided by the positive echoes in my life.

12. Identify the values you want to guide the next chapter of your life. Why is each value important to you and how can it shape your journey moving forward. What makes these values so significant in your story?

Example: I choose kindness as a guiding value because it shapes how I treat others and see the world. It's important in my story for creating positive relationships and a nurturing environment, key to my growth and happiness.

YOU ARE NOT YOUR TRAUMA HEALING JOURNAL

Confident	Excited	Calm	Appreciated	Afraid	Hurt	Angry
Determined	Happy	Content	Loved	Alarmed	Lonely	Annoyed
Encouraged	Hopeful	Focused	Supported	Anxious	Sad	Frustrated
Proud	Optimistic	Mindful	Valued	Fearful	Upset	Irritated
Supported	Overjoyed	Peaceful		Nervous		Mad
	Positive	Relaxed		Worried		

Notes_____

I live by values that uplift and guide my narrative positively.

13. Take a trip down memory lane and pick out a past memory. Now, try reimagining it by adding elements that fit with the story you want for yourself. How would this memory change to reflect the new narrative you're creating?

Example: I felt overlooked in a team meeting. I see myself speaking up confidently and being heard. This version aligns with my current narrative of becoming more assertive and valued in my professional life.

YOU ARE NOT YOUR TRAUMA HEALING JOURNAL

Confident	Excited	Calm	Appreciated	Afraid	Hurt	Angry
Determined	Happy	Content	Loved	Alarmed	Lonely	Annoyed
Encouraged	Hopeful	Focused	Supported	Anxious	Sad	Frustrated
Proud	Optimistic	Mindful	Valued	Fearful	Upset	Irritated
Supported	Overjoyed	Peaceful		Nervous		Mad
	Positive	Relaxed		Worried		

Notes _____

I have the creative liberty to reimagine and transform my past.

14. Who are the people who encourage you to be the author of your own story? How do they support you?

Example: My sister always encourages me to try new things, and my best friend is great at reminding me of my accomplishments.

YOU ARE NOT YOUR TRAUMA HEALING JOURNAL

Confident	Excited	Calm	Appreciated	Afraid	Hurt	Angry
Determined	Happy	Content	Loved	Alarmed	Lonely	Annoyed
Encouraged	Hopeful	Focused	Supported	Anxious	Sad	Frustrated
Proud	Optimistic	Mindful	Valued	Fearful	Upset	Irritated
Supported	Overjoyed	Peaceful		Nervous		Mad
	Positive	Relaxed		Worried		

Notes _____

I am supported and loved in the crafting of my new chapters.

15. Create a list of accomplishments, big or small, that you want to achieve in your new chapter.

Example: Run a 5K, learn to make pasta from scratch, and start a weekly gratitude journal.

YOU ARE NOT YOUR TRAUMA HEALING JOURNAL

_____
_____
_____
_____
_____
_____
_____
_____
_____
_____
_____
_____
_____
_____
_____
_____
_____
_____
_____
_____
_____
_____
_____
_____
_____
_____
_____
_____

Confident	Excited	Calm	Appreciated	Afraid	Hurt	Angry
Determined	Happy	Content	Loved	Alarmed	Lonely	Annoyed
Encouraged	Hopeful	Focused	Supported	Anxious	Sad	Frustrated
Proud	Optimistic	Mindful	Valued	Fearful	Upset	Irritated
Supported	Overjoyed	Peaceful		Nervous		Mad
	Positive	Relaxed		Worried		

☐ ☐ ☐ ☐ ☐ ☐ ☐ ☐

Notes_____
_____

I recognize and celebrate every achievement in my journey.

16. What are some simple, meaningful actions you can start today to shape your story in a positive direction?

Example: Today, I'll set aside 15 minutes for myself to read – it's a small step towards my goal of self-care.

YOU ARE NOT YOUR TRAUMA HEALING JOURNAL

Confident	Excited	Calm	Appreciated	Afraid	Hurt	Angry
Determined	Happy	Content	Loved	Alarmed	Lonely	Annoyed
Encouraged	Hopeful	Focused	Supported	Anxious	Sad	Frustrated
Proud	Optimistic	Mindful	Valued	Fearful	Upset	Irritated
Supported	Overjoyed	Peaceful		Nervous		Mad
	Positive	Relaxed		Worried		

Notes _____

Each step I take is purposeful and significant in shaping my narrative.

17. Describe a space where you feel safe and inspired to dream and where your creativity flows freely.

Example: My cozy reading nook at home, filled with soft pillows and surrounded by my favorite books.

YOU ARE NOT YOUR TRAUMA HEALING JOURNAL

Confident	Excited	Calm	Appreciated	Afraid	Hurt	Angry
Determined	Happy	Content	Loved	Alarmed	Lonely	Annoyed
Encouraged	Hopeful	Focused	Supported	Anxious	Sad	Frustrated
Proud	Optimistic	Mindful	Valued	Fearful	Upset	Irritated
Supported	Overjoyed	Peaceful		Nervous		Mad
	Positive	Relaxed		Worried		

Notes

I deserve safe spaces where I can dream and grow.

18. What's a phrase you can repeat to yourself to show kindness and encouragement as you navigate through writing your new life chapters?

Example: I am learning and growing every day, and I am proud of the progress I make.

_____
_____
_____
_____
_____
_____
_____
_____
_____
_____
_____
_____
_____
_____
_____
_____
_____
_____
_____
_____
_____
_____
_____
_____
_____
_____
_____
_____
_____

YOU ARE NOT YOUR TRAUMA HEALING JOURNAL

Confident	Excited	Calm	Appreciated	Afraid	Hurt	Angry
Determined	Happy	Content	Loved	Alarmed	Lonely	Annoyed
Encouraged	Hopeful	Focused	Supported	Anxious	Sad	Frustrated
Proud	Optimistic	Mindful	Valued	Fearful	Upset	Irritated
Supported	Overjoyed	Peaceful		Nervous		Mad
	Positive	Relaxed		Worried		
☐	☐	☐	☐	☐	☐	☐

Notes _____

I nurture myself with kindness and understanding.

19. Think about a moment in your life where you felt yourself growing or overcoming a challenge. How can you use that experience as a building block for the next chapter in your journey?

Example: I volunteered to lead a discussion at work, conquering my fear of public speaking. Despite the nerves, I felt empowered as I spoke, realizing the growth that comes from stepping out of my comfort zone.

YOU ARE NOT YOUR TRAUMA HEALING JOURNAL

Confident	Excited	Calm	Appreciated	Afraid	Hurt	Angry
Determined	Happy	Content	Loved	Alarmed	Lonely	Annoyed
Encouraged	Hopeful	Focused	Supported	Anxious	Sad	Frustrated
Proud	Optimistic	Mindful	Valued	Fearful	Upset	Irritated
Supported	Overjoyed	Peaceful		Nervous		Mad
	Positive	Relaxed		Worried		

Notes _____

I am continuously evolving, learning, and growing.

20. Think about the activities that make you genuinely happy. How can you prioritize these activities to incorporate them into your life more?

YOU ARE NOT YOUR TRAUMA HEALING JOURNAL

_____
_____
_____
_____
_____
_____
_____
_____
_____
_____
_____
_____
_____
_____
_____
_____
_____
_____
_____
_____
_____
_____
_____
_____
_____
_____
_____
_____
_____
_____
_____
_____

Confident	Excited	Calm	Appreciated	Afraid	Hurt	Angry
Determined	Happy	Content	Loved	Alarmed	Lonely	Annoyed
Encouraged	Hopeful	Focused	Supported	Anxious	Sad	Frustrated
Proud	Optimistic	Mindful	Valued	Fearful	Upset	Irritated
Supported	Overjoyed	Peaceful		Nervous		Mad
	Positive	Relaxed		Worried		
☐	☐	☐	☐	☐	☐	☐

Notes_____
_____

I deserve to engage in activities that bring me pure joy.

Part 3: Transformation

(Days 21-30)

Cultivating Change and Shaping New Narratives

This section signals your readiness to engage actively in the process of transformation. It is here that you start to reshape your narrative dynamically, identifying and releasing old patterns while cultivating new perspectives and stories that echo your true self and aspirations. It's a period of taking conscious steps towards a future you envision for yourself.

21. Visualize your life a year from now. What new stories have you added to the pages of your life?

Example: A year from now, I see myself in a job I love, spending quality time with family and friends, and taking a vacation abroad.

_____

YOU ARE NOT YOUR TRAUMA HEALING JOURNAL

Confident	Excited	Calm	Appreciated	Afraid	Hurt	Angry
Determined	Happy	Content	Loved	Alarmed	Lonely	Annoyed
Encouraged	Hopeful	Focused	Supported	Anxious	Sad	Frustrated
Proud	Optimistic	Mindful	Valued	Fearful	Upset	Irritated
Supported	Overjoyed	Peaceful		Nervous		Mad
	Positive	Relaxed		Worried		

Notes _____

I envision a narrative filled with positive stories and self-growth.

22. Imagine sketching out your desires, aspirations, and dreams for the narrative of your future. What would it look like on paper?

Confident	Excited	Calm	Appreciated	Afraid	Hurt	Angry
Determined	Happy	Content	Loved	Alarmed	Lonely	Annoyed
Encouraged	Hopeful	Focused	Supported	Anxious	Sad	Frustrated
Proud	Optimistic	Mindful	Valued	Fearful	Upset	Irritated
Supported	Overjoyed	Peaceful		Nervous		Mad
	Positive	Relaxed		Worried		
☐	☐	☐	☐	☐	☐	☐

Notes_____

My desires and dreams are valid and important.

23. Set personal milestones that you want to hit on your journey to reclaiming and reshaping your story.

Example: In the next six months, I aim to complete a professional certification, improve my fitness level, and volunteer regularly.

YOU ARE NOT YOUR TRAUMA HEALING JOURNAL

Confident	Excited	Calm	Appreciated	Afraid	Hurt	Angry
Determined	Happy	Content	Loved	Alarmed	Lonely	Annoyed
Encouraged	Hopeful	Focused	Supported	Anxious	Sad	Frustrated
Proud	Optimistic	Mindful	Valued	Fearful	Upset	Irritated
Supported	Overjoyed	Peaceful		Nervous		Mad
	Positive	Relaxed		Worried		

Notes _____

I set achievable milestones as a testament to my growth.

24. Imagine the legacy you want to leave. What stories do you want to write in the book of your life to create this legacy?

Example: I want to be remembered as someone who lifted others up and brought positivity to every situation.

YOU ARE NOT YOUR TRAUMA HEALING JOURNAL

Confident	Excited	Calm	Appreciated	Afraid	Hurt	Angry
Determined	Happy	Content	Loved	Alarmed	Lonely	Annoyed
Encouraged	Hopeful	Focused	Supported	Anxious	Sad	Frustrated
Proud	Optimistic	Mindful	Valued	Fearful	Upset	Irritated
Supported	Overjoyed	Peaceful		Nervous		Mad
	Positive	Relaxed		Worried		

Notes _____

I am building a legacy that reflects my true self.

25. What new habits can you begin to mark the beginning of new chapters in your life?

Example: Each morning, I'll write down three things I'm looking forward to in the day as a way to start my day on a positive note.

___

YOU ARE NOT YOUR TRAUMA HEALING JOURNAL

Confident	Excited	Calm	Appreciated	Afraid	Hurt	Angry
Determined	Happy	Content	Loved	Alarmed	Lonely	Annoyed
Encouraged	Hopeful	Focused	Supported	Anxious	Sad	Frustrated
Proud	Optimistic	Mindful	Valued	Fearful	Upset	Irritated
Supported	Overjoyed	Peaceful		Nervous		Mad
	Positive	Relaxed		Worried		

Notes _____

I create meaningful rituals that signify new beginnings.

26. Picture yourself a year from now. Describe what a day in your life looks like.

Example: A year from now, I start my day with yoga, work on my creative projects, and end the day cooking a new recipe with my family.

YOU ARE NOT YOUR TRAUMA HEALING JOURNAL

Confident	Excited	Calm	Appreciated	Afraid	Hurt	Angry
Determined	Happy	Content	Loved	Alarmed	Lonely	Annoyed
Encouraged	Hopeful	Focused	Supported	Anxious	Sad	Frustrated
Proud	Optimistic	Mindful	Valued	Fearful	Upset	Irritated
Supported	Overjoyed	Peaceful		Nervous		Mad
	Positive	Relaxed		Worried		
☐	☐	☐	☐	☐	☐	☐

Notes _____

I trust in the beautiful narrative unfolding for me.

27. What kind words or affirmations can you use to motivate yourself as you write new chapters in your life story?

Example: Your hard work is paying off. Keep pushing boundaries and exploring new horizons.

YOU ARE NOT YOUR TRAUMA HEALING JOURNAL

Confident	Excited	Calm	Appreciated	Afraid	Hurt	Angry
Determined	Happy	Content	Loved	Alarmed	Lonely	Annoyed
Encouraged	Hopeful	Focused	Supported	Anxious	Sad	Frustrated
Proud	Optimistic	Mindful	Valued	Fearful	Upset	Irritated
Supported	Overjoyed	Peaceful		Nervous		Mad
	Positive	Relaxed		Worried		

Notes_____

My inner dialogue is supportive and encouraging.

28. Choose symbols that represent your new chapter and describe what they mean to you.

Example: A rising sun would symbolize this new chapter. It represents hope, new beginnings, and the promise of a brighter future.

YOU ARE NOT YOUR TRAUMA HEALING JOURNAL

Confident	Excited	Calm	Appreciated	Afraid	Hurt	Angry
Determined	Happy	Content	Loved	Alarmed	Lonely	Annoyed
Encouraged	Hopeful	Focused	Supported	Anxious	Sad	Frustrated
Proud	Optimistic	Mindful	Valued	Fearful	Upset	Irritated
Supported	Overjoyed	Peaceful		Nervous		Mad
	Positive	Relaxed		Worried		

Notes

I choose symbols that empower and represent me well.

29. Create clear, achievable goals for healing and growth that you can focus on as you start this new chapter in your life.

YOU ARE NOT YOUR TRAUMA HEALING JOURNAL

Confident	Excited	Calm	Appreciated	Afraid	Hurt	Angry
Determined	Happy	Content	Loved	Alarmed	Lonely	Annoyed
Encouraged	Hopeful	Focused	Supported	Anxious	Sad	Frustrated
Proud	Optimistic	Mindful	Valued	Fearful	Upset	Irritated
Supported	Overjoyed	Peaceful		Nervous		Mad
	Positive	Relaxed		Worried		

Notes _____

I set achievable goals that align with my vision for myself.

30. What are some new, positive experiences or moments you're grateful for? Make it a habit to journal about them regularly.

YOU ARE NOT YOUR TRAUMA HEALING JOURNAL

Confident	Excited	Calm	Appreciated	Afraid	Hurt	Angry
Determined	Happy	Content	Loved	Alarmed	Lonely	Annoyed
Encouraged	Hopeful	Focused	Supported	Anxious	Sad	Frustrated
Proud	Optimistic	Mindful	Valued	Fearful	Upset	Irritated
Supported	Overjoyed	Peaceful		Nervous		Mad
	Positive	Relaxed		Worried		

Notes _____

I embrace the present, cherishing the positive moments life offers.

Part 4: Blossoming

(Days 31-40)

Embracing Your Renewed Self

It's time to blossom, to bring to fruition all the insights and growth cultivated during this journey. In this stage, you will witness the beautiful unfolding of your renewed self, a time to celebrate the resilience, the learning, and the blossoming of a self more in tune with its core essence, dreams, and desires.

31. How do you envision yourself stepping into the role of the hero in your story?

YOU ARE NOT YOUR TRAUMA HEALING JOURNAL

Confident	Excited	Calm	Appreciated	Afraid	Hurt	Angry
Determined	Happy	Content	Loved	Alarmed	Lonely	Annoyed
Encouraged	Hopeful	Focused	Supported	Anxious	Sad	Frustrated
Proud	Optimistic	Mindful	Valued	Fearful	Upset	Irritated
Supported	Overjoyed	Peaceful		Nervous		Mad
	Positive	Relaxed		Worried		

Notes _____

I am the hero of my story, navigating through life with courage.

32. How do you anticipate using challenging experiences as learning opportunities to shape your future narratives positively?

YOU ARE NOT YOUR TRAUMA HEALING JOURNAL

Confident	Excited	Calm	Appreciated	Afraid	Hurt	Angry
Determined	Happy	Content	Loved	Alarmed	Lonely	Annoyed
Encouraged	Hopeful	Focused	Supported	Anxious	Sad	Frustrated
Proud	Optimistic	Mindful	Valued	Fearful	Upset	Irritated
Supported	Overjoyed	Peaceful		Nervous		Mad
	Positive	Relaxed		Worried		

Notes_____

Every experience is a learning opportunity, guiding my growth.

33. Imagine how practicing forgiveness will shape your future narratives positively as you move forward on your journey of personal growth and healing.

YOU ARE NOT YOUR TRAUMA HEALING JOURNAL

Confident	Excited	Calm	Appreciated	Afraid	Hurt	Angry
Determined	Happy	Content	Loved	Alarmed	Lonely	Annoyed
Encouraged	Hopeful	Focused	Supported	Anxious	Sad	Frustrated
Proud	Optimistic	Mindful	Valued	Fearful	Upset	Irritated
Supported	Overjoyed	Peaceful		Nervous		Mad
	Positive	Relaxed		Worried		

Notes _____

I embrace forgiveness, fostering peace and forward movement in my narrative.

34. Describe your spirit using words that show your resilience and strength. How do you see these qualities helping you grow and thrive in the future?

YOU ARE NOT YOUR TRAUMA HEALING JOURNAL

Confident	Excited	Calm	Appreciated	Afraid	Hurt	Angry
Determined	Happy	Content	Loved	Alarmed	Lonely	Annoyed
Encouraged	Hopeful	Focused	Supported	Anxious	Sad	Frustrated
Proud	Optimistic	Mindful	Valued	Fearful	Upset	Irritated
Supported	Overjoyed	Peaceful		Nervous		Mad
	Positive	Relaxed		Worried		

Notes

I am resilient, with a spirit that thrives through challenges.

35. Think about people who inspire the new chapter of your life. What qualities do they have that you admire, and how can you incorporate these qualities into your future self?

YOU ARE NOT YOUR TRAUMA HEALING JOURNAL

Confident	Excited	Calm	Appreciated	Afraid	Hurt	Angry
Determined	Happy	Content	Loved	Alarmed	Lonely	Annoyed
Encouraged	Hopeful	Focused	Supported	Anxious	Sad	Frustrated
Proud	Optimistic	Mindful	Valued	Fearful	Upset	Irritated
Supported	Overjoyed	Peaceful		Nervous		Mad
	Positive	Relaxed		Worried		

Notes _____

I embody the qualities I admire in others, shaping my unique narrative.

36. Think of a fear that's been holding you back and turn it into a fictional story. How can reimagining this fear help you embrace your future with more confidence and strength?

YOU ARE NOT YOUR TRAUMA HEALING JOURNAL

Confident	Excited	Calm	Appreciated	Afraid	Hurt	Angry
Determined	Happy	Content	Loved	Alarmed	Lonely	Annoyed
Encouraged	Hopeful	Focused	Supported	Anxious	Sad	Frustrated
Proud	Optimistic	Mindful	Valued	Fearful	Upset	Irritated
Supported	Overjoyed	Peaceful		Nervous		Mad
	Positive	Relaxed		Worried		

Notes_____

I have the power to transform fear into a story of strength.

37. Picture how you see yourself growing and changing in the future. Draw or describe your self-portrait as you move through the different chapters of your life.

YOU ARE NOT YOUR TRAUMA HEALING JOURNAL

Confident	Excited	Calm	Appreciated	Afraid	Hurt	Angry
Determined	Happy	Content	Loved	Alarmed	Lonely	Annoyed
Encouraged	Hopeful	Focused	Supported	Anxious	Sad	Frustrated
Proud	Optimistic	Mindful	Valued	Fearful	Upset	Irritated
Supported	Overjoyed	Peaceful		Nervous		Mad
	Positive	Relaxed		Worried		

Notes _____

I celebrate the evolving portrait of myself, showcasing my growth through phases.

38. Reflect on the growth you've experienced. Write affirmations that celebrate your progress and inspire you to continue blossoming into your best self.

Confident	Excited	Calm	Appreciated	Afraid	Hurt	Angry
Determined	Happy	Content	Loved	Alarmed	Lonely	Annoyed
Encouraged	Hopeful	Focused	Supported	Anxious	Sad	Frustrated
Proud	Optimistic	Mindful	Valued	Fearful	Upset	Irritated
Supported	Overjoyed	Peaceful		Nervous		Mad
	Positive	Relaxed		Worried		

Notes _____

I affirm my worth and potential daily.

39. Create a visual diary of moments that symbolize new beginnings and positive experiences. How can capturing these moments help you continue to grow and embrace your renewed self?

YOU ARE NOT YOUR TRAUMA HEALING JOURNAL

Confident	Excited	Calm	Appreciated	Afraid	Hurt	Angry
Determined	Happy	Content	Loved	Alarmed	Lonely	Annoyed
Encouraged	Hopeful	Focused	Supported	Anxious	Sad	Frustrated
Proud	Optimistic	Mindful	Valued	Fearful	Upset	Irritated
Supported	Overjoyed	Peaceful		Nervous		Mad
	Positive	Relaxed		Worried		

Notes _____

I document my journey, valuing every step towards positive change.

40. As your journey comes to a close, write a letter to yourself, celebrating the journey you've undertaken to shape your narrative beyond trauma.

YOU ARE NOT YOUR TRAUMA HEALING JOURNAL

Confident	Excited	Calm	Appreciated	Afraid	Hurt	Angry
Determined	Happy	Content	Loved	Alarmed	Lonely	Annoyed
Encouraged	Hopeful	Focused	Supported	Anxious	Sad	Frustrated
Proud	Optimistic	Mindful	Valued	Fearful	Upset	Irritated
Supported	Overjoyed	Peaceful		Nervous		Mad
	Positive	Relaxed		Worried		
☐	☐	☐	☐	☐	☐	☐

Notes_____

I honor and celebrate the resilient journey I have embarked upon.

After the 40 Days
Stepping into Post-Traumatic Growth

Congratulations you did it—you completed your 40-day journey! You've made incredible strides in writing the next chapters in your life story and envisioning a future that moves beyond the shadows of the past. As you shift from reflection and vision to living your new story, you're stepping into the transformative phase of Post-Traumatic Growth.

Here's how to embrace this new phase and start living out the chapters you've envisioned:

1. **Reflect on Your Journey**: Take some time to look back through your journal. Notice the changes from where you started to where you are now. Highlight the key insights and the dreams that excite you the most.
2. **Create an Action Plan**: Turn those dreams into actionable steps. Break your goals into smaller, manageable parts, and set achievable timelines.
3. **Set Daily Intentions**: Start each day with a goal that reflects your new story. It could be something simple like a daily moment of gratitude or something more extensive like moving towards a new job.
4. **Embrace New Habits**: Make the positive habits and rituals from your journaling a regular part of your day. Whether it's a morning walk, creative time, or a new exercise routine, incorporate these into your daily life.
5. **Lean on Your Support Network**: Share your new journey with friends, family, or a support group. Let them know how they can be part of this new chapter with you.
6. **Keep the Dialogue Going**: Don't stop journaling. Your structured 40 days might be over, but the conversation with yourself is ongoing. Regular check-ins with your journal can help keep you on track with your new path.
7. **Celebrate Every Step**: Recognize and celebrate each small win. These moments of celebration are vital to staying motivated and recognizing your progress.
8. **Stay Open and Adaptable**: As you walk this new path, stay

open to life's unexpected turns. Your story will evolve, so be ready to adapt and grow.
9. **Keep Learning**: Actively seek knowledge and skills that align with your new narrative. Whether through books, classes, or conversations with mentors, keep feeding your mind.
10. **Give Back**: Think about ways to use your experiences to help others. Often, supporting others in their journeys can reinforce and deepen our growth.

As you step into your Post-Traumatic Growth, remember that the end of this structured journaling is not the conclusion of your journey but the beginning of a powerful transformation. You're now equipped with insights and tools to bring your vision to life. Embrace this change, step confidently into your new narrative, and live out your story with courage, hope, and resilience. This next phase is about thriving, not just surviving, and using your experiences as a foundation for a rich, fulfilling life.

Welcome to your journey of Post-Traumatic Growth!

Understanding and Navigating Your Transformation

As you progress from this initial 40-day journey, you're entering a critical phase of your healing process: understanding and embracing Post-Traumatic Growth (PTG). This phase goes beyond merely surviving trauma, this step is about thriving afterward, using your experiences as a springboard for profound personal growth.

In this phase, you'll shift your focus from exploring the depths of your inner world to understanding how these experiences have prepared you for positive change. You'll learn to recognize and nurture the seeds of growth that have taken root in the soil of your struggles. This part of your journey is about seeing how your experiences have expanded your capacity for empathy, deepened your understanding of yourself and others, and reshaped your view of life.

Despite the name, Post-Traumatic Growth isn't about the trauma itself but about how you respond. It refers to the way you've grown and your ability to find new meaning from your experiences with trauma. PTG can show up in different ways, including a greater appreciation of life, improved personal relationships, increased personal strength, new possibilities for your life, and spiritual growth.

Exploring the Essence of Post-Traumatic Growth

PTG represents the positive psychological change resulting from struggling with challenging life circumstances. It manifests in five key areas:

1. **New Appreciation for Life**: You might begin valuing life more intensely, feeling a heightened sense of gratitude, and savoring everyday pleasures you previously overlooked.
2. **Improved Relationships**: Trauma can deepen your empathy and connection with others, leading to more meaningful and compassionate relationships.
3. **Personal Strength**: You may discover an inner resilience and strength you didn't know you had, boosting your confidence in overcoming future challenges.
4. **New Paths and Possibilities**: PTG often shifts your perspective,

opening doors to new opportunities and interests you might not have considered before. This change can help you reevaluate your life goals and explore paths that align more closely with who you are now.
5. **Spiritual Development**: Many find their experiences lead to a deeper exploration of spiritual beliefs or a newfound sense of spirituality.

Cultivating Post-Traumatic Growth in Your Life

PTG doesn't happen automatically or overnight. It's a process that involves active engagement in self-reflection, understanding, and redefining your life values and goals. Here are some ways to nurture PTG:

- **Mindful Reflection**: Regularly practice mindfulness and self-reflection to stay aware of your growth journey.
- **Pursue Meaningful Activities**: Engage in activities that align with your values and provide a sense of purpose, like creative hobbies, volunteering, or spiritual practices.
- **Build and Maintain Relationships**: Cultivate strong support networks and deepen your relationships through open communication and shared experiences.
- **Embrace New Opportunities**: Be open to exploring new avenues in life, whether career changes, educational pursuits, or personal interests sparked by your journey.
- **Stay Hopeful and Goal-Oriented**: Set realistic and achievable goals for yourself and maintain an optimistic outlook.

Integrating Post-Traumatic Growth into Your Journey

Recognizing and integrating PTG into your life is a dynamic and ongoing process. As you continue your journey, use the insights and strengths you've gained to shape a life that reflects your growth. In this phase focus on turning your experiences into a force for positive change, allowing you to build a life narrative rich with resilience, purpose, and fulfillment.

Embrace this phase of Post-Traumatic Growth as a chance to

transform your trauma into triumph and create a future that's full of possibilities and joy.

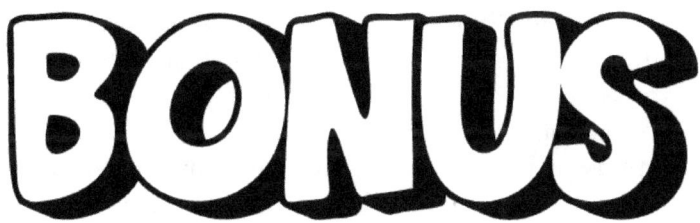

Charting Your Path Forward

Setting Your Healing Goals

As you turn the final pages of this book, it's time to channel the insights and dreams you've nurtured over the past 40 days into concrete goals for your ongoing healing journey. These goals are your personal milestones on the road to a future where you survive and thrive. Here's a guide to setting your healing goals:

1. **Reflect on Your 40-Day Journey**: Look back at the thoughts, dreams, and visions you recorded in your journal. What themes or aspirations stood out? What have you discovered about yourself and your path forward?
2. **Envision a Future Informed by Your Journaling**: Think about the future you've been shaping in your journal. Imagine what this future looks like now that you've spent 40 days focusing on your growth and healing. How does this vision feel, and what does it include?
3. **Identify Your Focus Areas**: Based on your reflections and envisioned future, pinpoint specific areas you want to focus on for further healing and growth. This could involve enhancing personal relationships, pursuing new career goals, or developing self-care practices.
4. **Set Specific, Achievable Goals**: Make your goals tangible and realistic. Instead of vague aspirations, choose actionable objectives that directly contribute to your healing.
5. **Break Down Your Goals**: Break each goal into smaller, manageable, and less overwhelming steps. For example, if your goal is to build more meaningful connections, one step could be to reach out to a friend or family member weekly.
6. **Write Down Your Goals**: There's power in writing your goals down. Keep them where you can review them often, like the journal you've been using or a spot in your home you see daily.
7. **Regularly Review and Adjust**: Your goals aren't set in stone. As you grow and evolve, so too can your goals. Regularly check in with yourself and adjust your goals as needed to align with your journey.
8. **Celebrate Each Step Forward**: Recognize and celebrate your progress. Every little step you take is a testament to your

strength and commitment to your healing.

Your goals are an extension of the transformative work you've begun with this book. They represent your commitment to yourself and your future—a future that's been carefully crafted through 40 days of introspection and dreaming. As you move forward, remember that each goal, each step, is a part of your larger journey toward a life defined by resilience, healing, and fulfillment.

Create Your Own Healing Goals

Setting clear and meaningful goals will be your roadmap as you shift into this next phase of your journey. Use the space on the following pages to articulate these goals. Alongside each goal, there's additional guidance to ensure your goals are well-defined, inspiring, and achievable.

Goal-Setting Format

1. **Goal Title**: Give your goal a motivating title that instantly reminds you of what you're working towards.
2. **Inspiration from Journaling**: Reflect on your 40-day journey. How did your journaling inspire this particular goal? Write down specific thoughts, dreams, or insights from your journal related to this goal.
3. **Detailed Description**: Elaborate on what this goal means to you. Be as specific as possible about what achieving this goal looks like.
4. **Motivation**: Why is this goal important to you? Understanding your motivation will keep you driven, especially during challenging times.
5. **Action Steps**: Break down the goal into smaller, manageable action steps. List out these steps clearly.
6. **Timeline**: Set a realistic timeline for each action step. Having a timeline helps in tracking your progress and maintaining your momentum.
7. **Resources Needed**: Identify any resources or support you might need. Consider resources like books, support groups, tools, or people.
8. **Progress Checkpoints**: Establish dates or intervals to review your progress. This will help you stay on track and make necessary adjustments.
9. **Celebration Plan**: Decide how you will celebrate achieving this goal. Celebrations are important for recognizing your hard work and success.

Additional Guidance

- ✓ **Be Realistic**: Set goals that are challenging yet achievable. Unrealistic goals can be discouraging.
- ✓ **Stay Flexible**: Be open to modifying your goals as you progress. Flexibility is key to adapting to life's changes and your growth.
- ✓ **Seek Support**: Don't hesitate to share your goals with trusted friends or family members who can offer support and encouragement.
- ✓ **Visualize Success**: Regularly visualize yourself achieving your goals. This positive visualization can be a powerful motivator.
- ✓ **Practice Self-Compassion**: Be kind to yourself if progress is slower than expected. Healing is not linear, and every small step counts.
- ✓ **Stay Connected to Your Why**: Regularly remind yourself why these goals are important. This connection will keep your motivation strong.

Use the space on the following pages to create your own healing goals. This structured approach and guidance will equip you with a clear and actionable plan for your healing journey. Each goal you set is a step towards a future where your trauma no longer holds you back but propels you forward to grow. Remember, these goals are essential to the life you want to create for yourself.

Revisit and update this template as you progress, adapting it to fit your journey's evolving nature.

My Healing Goals
Complete for each goal.

Goal Title: _____

Inspiration from Journaling: _____
_____
_____
_____

Detailed Description: _____
_____
_____
_____
_____
_____
_____

Motivation: _____
_____
_____
_____

Action Steps: _____
_____
_____
_____
_____
_____

Timeline for Each Step: _____
_____
_____
_____
_____
_____

Resources Needed: _____
_____
_____

Progress Checkpoints: _____
_____
_____
_____
_____
_____

Celebration Plan:
_____
_____
_____
_____

Additional Notes: _____
_____
_____
_____
_____
_____
_____
_____
_____
_____
_____
_____
_____
_____

Goal Title: _____

Inspiration from Journaling: _____
_____
_____
_____

Detailed Description: _____
_____
_____
_____
_____
_____
_____

Motivation: _____
_____
_____
_____

Action Steps: _____
_____
_____
_____
_____

Timeline for Each Step: _____
_____
_____
_____
_____
_____

Resources Needed: _____
_____
_____

Progress Checkpoints: _____
_____
_____
_____
_____
_____

Celebration Plan:
_____
_____
_____
_____
_____

Additional Notes: _____
_____
_____
_____
_____
_____
_____
_____
_____
_____
_____
_____
_____
_____
_____

Goal Title: _____

Inspiration from Journaling: _____
_____
_____
_____

Detailed Description: _____
_____
_____
_____
_____
_____
_____
_____

Motivation: _____
_____
_____
_____

Action Steps: _____
_____
_____
_____
_____
_____

Timeline for Each Step: _____
_____
_____
_____
_____
_____

Resources Needed: _____

Progress Checkpoints: _____

_____

Celebration Plan:

_____

Additional Notes: _____

Goal Title: _____

Inspiration from Journaling: _____
_____
_____
_____

Detailed Description: _____
_____
_____
_____
_____
_____
_____

Motivation: _____
_____
_____

Action Steps: _____
_____
_____
_____
_____
_____

Timeline for Each Step: _____
_____
_____
_____
_____
_____

Resources Needed: _____

Progress Checkpoints: _____

Celebration Plan:

Additional Notes: _____

Goal Title: _____

Inspiration from Journaling: _____
_____
_____
_____

Detailed Description: _____
_____
_____
_____
_____
_____
_____
_____

Motivation: _____
_____
_____
_____

Action Steps: _____
_____
_____
_____
_____
_____
_____

Timeline for Each Step: _____
_____
_____
_____
_____
_____

Resources Needed: _____

Progress Checkpoints: _____

Celebration Plan:

Additional Notes: _____

Goal Title: _____

Inspiration from Journaling: _____
_____
_____
_____

Detailed Description: _____
_____
_____
_____
_____
_____
_____

Motivation: _____
_____
_____
_____

Action Steps: _____
_____
_____
_____
_____
_____

Timeline for Each Step: _____
_____
_____
_____
_____
_____

Resources Needed: _____

Progress Checkpoints: _____

Celebration Plan:

Additional Notes: _____

Goal Title: _____

Inspiration from Journaling: _____
_____
_____
_____

Detailed Description: _____
_____
_____
_____
_____
_____
_____

Motivation: _____
_____
_____
_____

Action Steps: _____
_____
_____
_____
_____
_____

Timeline for Each Step: _____
_____
_____
_____
_____
_____

Resources Needed: _____

Progress Checkpoints: _____

Celebration Plan:

Additional Notes: _____

Goal Title: _____

Inspiration from Journaling: _____
_____
_____
_____

Detailed Description: _____
_____
_____
_____
_____
_____
_____

Motivation: _____
_____
_____
_____

Action Steps: _____
_____
_____
_____
_____
_____

Timeline for Each Step: _____
_____
_____
_____
_____
_____

Resources Needed: _____

Progress Checkpoints: _____

Celebration Plan:

Additional Notes: _____

Goal Title: _____

Inspiration from Journaling: _____
_____
_____
_____

Detailed Description: _____
_____
_____
_____
_____
_____
_____

Motivation: _____
_____
_____
_____

Action Steps: _____
_____
_____
_____
_____
_____
_____

Timeline for Each Step: _____
_____
_____
_____
_____
_____

Resources Needed: _____

_____
_____

Progress Checkpoints: _____
_____
_____
_____
_____
_____

Celebration Plan:
_____
_____
_____
_____
_____

Additional Notes: _____
_____
_____
_____
_____
_____
_____
_____
_____
_____
_____
_____
_____
_____
_____

Goal Title: _____

Inspiration from Journaling: _____
_____
_____
_____

Detailed Description: _____
_____
_____
_____
_____
_____
_____
_____

Motivation: _____
_____
_____
_____

Action Steps: _____
_____
_____
_____
_____
_____

Timeline for Each Step: _____
_____
_____
_____
_____
_____

Resources Needed: _____

Progress Checkpoints:

Celebration Plan:

Additional Notes:

Goal Title: _____

Inspiration from Journaling: _____
_____
_____
_____

Detailed Description: _____
_____
_____
_____
_____
_____
_____

Motivation: _____
_____
_____
_____

Action Steps: _____
_____
_____
_____
_____
_____

Timeline for Each Step: _____
_____
_____
_____
_____
_____

Resources Needed: _____

_____

_____

Progress Checkpoints: _____

_____

_____

_____

_____

_____

Celebration Plan:

_____

_____

_____

_____

Additional Notes: _____

_____

_____

_____

_____

_____

_____

_____

_____

_____

_____

_____

_____

_____

New Narrative Ground Rules

You're on the brink of something new! Gearing up for a journey to uncharted territories in your life. To navigate this adventure successfully, you need to establish some ground rules – consider these your guide for the journey ahead. Let's call them your New Narrative Ground Rules.

These ground rules are your personal guidelines for navigating the future and propelling you forward into a life where you thrive. They are non-negotiable, the fundamental principles that will help you stay aligned with your vision and values. Here are the steps to create them:

1. **Pause and Reflect**: Look back on this journey you've taken over the past 40 days. What moments made you feel alive? What lessons do you want to carry forward?
2. **Identify Your Key Lessons**: From the insights you've gathered, identify the core principles you want to guide you. These are the seeds for your ground rules.
3. **Dream Big, Start Small**: Think about the life you're stepping into. Break down your big dreams into tangible, guiding principles.
4. **Pen to Paper**: Time to make it real. Write down these ground rules. Keep them somewhere you'll see daily – a constant reminder of your path forward.
5. **Live by Them**: Transform these rules into your daily mantras. Embrace them, believe in their power, and let them become a part of who you are.

Examples to Get You Started:

Rule #1: This rule is about finding joy.
Example: "I will find one thing that makes me smile every day, no matter how small."

Rule #2: This rule is about growth.
Example: "Each week, I'll explore something new, whether it's a skill, book, or place."

Rule #3: This rule is about resilience.
Example: "I'll recognize my struggles but focus on solutions and learning from them."

Rule #4: This rule is about connection.
Example "I'll make an effort to connect with a loved one weekly, nurturing my relationships."

Add as many rules as you feel necessary to guide you toward the life you envision.

My Ground Rules

Remember, these ground rules are your personal guide to ensuring that you continue moving forward with purpose and positivity. Embrace them, adapt them as needed, and let them be the foundation of your new, empowered narrative.

These rules are your commitment to a life defined by your terms, your growth, and your joy. It's important to set boundaries that protect your progress and prevent you from slipping back into old patterns. These rules are your declaration: "This is my life, and I'm steering it towards my dreams with intention and heart."

Final Thoughts

As you close this book, remember that your journey doesn't end here. You've laid the groundwork for a future filled with endless possibilities. Keep this momentum going, continue to write your story, and embrace every chapter with courage and hope.

Thank you for trusting this journal to be a part of your healing journey. May you continue to thrive, live boldly, and inspire others with your strength and grace.

With deepest gratitude,

Harriet M. Harris, MBA

ABOUT THE AUTHOR

Harriet M. Harris, MBA, is a speaker, author, trauma-informed coach, and the compassionate voice behind You Are Not Your Trauma podcast. She is also the founder of You Are Not Your Trauma Inc., an non-profit dedicated to empowering individuals to heal from trauma by helping them realize they are not defined by their traumas. Through this platform, Harriet provides resources, and a supportive community focused on changing the stigma around trauma and healing. Her goal is to help individuals choose healing over hurting.

Harriet's mission is to foster healing and empower individuals—particularly women—to understand that their past experiences do not define them. She guides her clients and audiences to shed limiting beliefs, facilitating transformative change in both life and business. She believes that those that have experienced trauma, survived to thrive and that everyone has the potential to live a fulfilling life beyond their past experiences.

Understanding that one cannot reach their full potential without addressing the emotional and mental scars of trauma, Harriet employs a holistic approach in her coaching. She integrates personal development and healing methodologies into her unique coaching style. Her programs focus on implementing effective systems, processes, and accountability structures, creating an environment that nurtures professional and personal growth.

Harriet is a sought-after public speaker on topics such as trauma healing, the importance of self-kindness, self-care, and overcoming self-imposed limitations. Her empowering message resonates deeply with those ready to take the first steps toward healing and living a life of limitless possibilities.

CONNECT WITH ME

Congratulations again on taking this journey of healing and empowerment. I am so proud of you! I would love for you to connect with me! Here are all the ways you can connect, access resources, and continue your journey with me:

Check out You Are Not Your Trauma™ Podcast
Tune in to the "You Are Not Your Trauma™ podcast, where we explore resilience, emotional healing, and the journey from surviving trauma to embracing a limitless future.

Download the You Are Not Your Trauma™ App
Access exclusive content, community support, and personalized resources right from your phone. Download the You Are Not Your Trauma™ app:

Explore the You Are Not Your Trauma™ Resource Guide
Find comprehensive resources to support your healing journey. From articles and videos to worksheets and exercises, the You Are Not Your Trauma™ Resource Guide has tools to support you on your healing journey.
Grab your copy here: resourceguide.youarenotyourtrauma.com

Grab a signed copy of Stop Stopping Your Success
Unlock actionable insights and strategies to overcome barriers and achieve a fulfilling life. Order your copy here: book.stopstoppingyoursuccess.com

Contact Me
For speaking engagements, coaching inquiries, or to simply reach out, contact me at: contact@harrietmharris.com

Thank you for being a part of this journey.

www.ingramcontent.com/pod-product-compliance
Lightning Source LLC
Chambersburg PA
CBHW060503030426
42337CB00015B/1712